A 6-Minutes Fitness For 60+ (Isometric Exercises)

A Comprehensive Guide To Utilizing Isometric Exercises Effectively Maximizing Muscle Growth And Preventing Muscle Loss

Brayan Reynolds

Table of Contents

CHAPTER ONE
Introduction To Isometric Exercises

Isometric exercises are a form of strength training where the muscle contracts but doesn't change length, meaning there's no joint movement or visible muscle contraction. Instead, you hold a position against resistance, like pushing against an immovable object or holding a position statically.

These exercises engage specific muscles or groups without movement. Imagine pushing against a wall or holding a plank position—those are classic isometric exercises. They're great for building strength, enhancing stability, and improving muscle endurance. Plus, they're convenient; you can do them anywhere without any equipment.

Benefits and Advantages

Isometric training offers several benefits:

Strength Gains: Isometric exercises engage muscle fibers, leading to increased strength. They target specific muscle groups intensely, promoting strength gains in those areas.

Improved Joint Stability: Holding isometric positions can enhance joint stability by strengthening the muscles around them. This helps in injury prevention and supports joint health.

Time Efficiency: Isometric exercises can be done quickly and don't require a lot of space or equipment, making them a convenient choice for busy schedules.

Lower Risk of Injury: As there's no joint movement, isometric exercises typically have a lower risk of causing injury compared to dynamic exercises involving joint motion.

Improved Muscle Endurance: Regularly incorporating isometric exercises into a workout routine can improve muscle endurance, allowing you to hold positions for longer periods.

Accessible for Various Fitness Levels: Isometric exercises can be adapted to suit different fitness levels, from beginners to advanced athletes, by adjusting the duration and intensity of the holds.

Convenient for Rehabilitation: Isometric exercises are often used in physical therapy to help regain strength and mobility after an injury due to their low impact nature.

Isometric Exercises by Body Regions (Upper Body Isometrics)

Some isometric exercises targeting the upper body are:

Push-Up Variations: Isometrically holding different positions within a push-up can engage various muscle groups.

Mid-Position Hold: Pause halfway down in a push-up, holding the position for a set duration.

Top Position Hold: Hold at the top of a push-up with arms fully extended.

Static Hold for Chest and Arms:

Wall Press: Stand facing a wall with your arms bent at 90 degrees, press into the wall, and hold the position.

Isometric Chest Squeeze: Hold a yoga block, ball, or a towel between your hands in front of your chest and press inward while holding.

Isometric Rows:

Towel or Band Rows: Loop a towel or resistance band around a stable object, hold each end, and pull the towel/band toward you, engaging your back muscles while holding the contraction.

Lower Body Isometrics

Some effective lower body isometric exercises are as follows:

Wall Sit Progressions:

Classic Wall Sit: Sit against a wall with your knees bent at a 90-degree angle, thighs parallel to the floor, and hold this position.

Single-Leg Wall Sit: Similar to the classic wall sit, but with one leg raised, challenging one leg at a time.

Wall Sit with Calf Raises: Combine a wall sit with calf raises by lifting your heels while maintaining the seated position.

Isometric Step-Ups:

Elevated Surface Holds: Place one foot on an elevated surface (step or sturdy platform), lift your body up, and hold the top position with your leg at a 90-degree angle.

Isometric Lunge Hold: Similar to a step-up, but holding a lunge position with the front leg at a 90-degree angle.

Isometric Deadlift Holds:

Barbell or Dumbbell Hold: Hold a barbell or dumbbells at the top of a deadlift movement, keeping your body upright and holding the contraction in your hamstrings, glutes, and lower back.

Core Isometrics

Core isometric exercises are fantastic for building abdominal and trunk strength. Here are some effective options:

Plank Variations:

Standard Plank: Maintain a push-up position with your body in a straight line from head to heels, supporting yourself on your forearms and toes.

Side Plank: Support your body sideways on one forearm and the side of your foot, keeping your body in a straight line, engaging the obliques.

Plank with Arm/Leg Lift: From a standard plank position, lift one arm or leg and hold the position, engaging the core muscles to maintain stability.

Russian Twists Hold:

Weighted Russian Twist Hold: Sit on the floor, lean back slightly, lift your legs off the ground, and hold while twisting your torso from side to side while holding a weight or keeping your hands clasped together.

Hollow Body Hold:

Supine Hollow Hold: Lie on your back, engage your core, lift your legs and shoulders off the ground, creating a "hollow" shape with your body, and hold the position.

These exercises focus on engaging and strengthening the core muscles, helping to improve stability, posture, and overall strength in the abdominal and trunk region.

Dynamic Isometric Movements

Dynamic isometric movements combine the stability of isometric contractions with the dynamic nature of movement, providing an effective way to train explosiveness and strength. There exists different types, they are:

Isometric-Ballistic Combinations:

Plyometric Push-Ups: Perform a standard push-up but explosively push yourself up so your hands leave the ground. At the top, hold an isometric contraction before descending into the next push-up.

Isometric Squat Jumps: Lower into a squat position, explode up into a jump, and upon landing, hold a squat position for a brief isometric contraction before jumping again.

Explosive Isometric Training:

Isometric Medicine Ball Throws: Hold a medicine ball in an isometric hold, then explosively throw it against a wall or to a partner.

Isometric Band Pulls: Hold a resistance band in a fixed position and perform explosive pulls against the resistance while holding the isometric position.

Isometric Contractions with Movement:

Iso-Holds during Lunges: Perform lunges and pause at the lowest point of the movement, holding an isometric contraction before returning to the starting position.

Isometric Holds with Leg Raises: During leg raises, pause at the top of the movement and hold the position briefly before lowering your legs back down.

These dynamic isometric movements combine the benefits of explosive movements with the stability and strength gained from isometric contractions.

CHAPTER TWO

Isometric Partner Workouts

Partner workouts can add a fun and interactive element to isometric exercises. Here are some partner-based isometric exercises:

Partner-Assisted Isometric Holds:

Partner Wall Sit: Both partners sit back-to-back against a wall, supporting each other's weight while holding a wall sit position.

Plank High-Five: Both partners assume a plank position facing each other, and while maintaining the plank, alternate raising one hand to high-five each other.

Dual Resistance Band Exercises:

Band Resistance Squat Hold: Both partners hold opposite ends of a resistance band while performing squats, creating resistance for each other.

Partner Band Rows: Face each other, each holding one end of a resistance band, and perform rows while providing resistance to each other's movements.

Synchronized Isometric Movements:

Mirror Image Planks: Partners face each other in a plank position and mirror each other's movements, engaging in synchronized plank variations.

Side Plank High-Five: Both partners assume a side plank position facing each other and reach under their bodies to high-five with the bottom hand.

These partner-based isometric exercises not only provide a unique way to challenge each other's strength but also foster teamwork and motivation.

Isometric Training with Equipment

Isometric training with various equipment can add versatility and intensity to your workouts. Here are ways to incorporate isometric exercises using specific equipment:

TRX Isometric Variations:

TRX Plank Hold: Assume a plank position with your feet in the TRX straps, holding the plank while the straps add instability, engaging more muscles for stability.

TRX Row Hold: Perform a row with the TRX straps and hold the end position, engaging your back muscles isometrically.

Kettlebell Isometric Holds:

Kettlebell Goblet Squat Hold: Hold a kettlebell at chest level while in a squat position, maintaining the hold to engage leg and core muscles.

Kettlebell Overhead Hold: Hold a kettlebell overhead, engaging your shoulders, arms, and core to stabilize the weight.

Isometric Exercises using Resistance Bands:

Band Pull-Apart Hold: Hold a resistance band at chest level and pull it apart, holding the end position to engage the shoulders and upper back.

Band Isometric Squats: Place a resistance band above your knees, assume a squat position, and hold it isometrically against the band's resistance.

These equipment-based isometric exercises can be adjusted in difficulty by modifying the weight or resistance, making them adaptable to different fitness levels.

Advanced Isometric Training

Advanced isometric training introduces challenging variations that require significant strength and balance. Here are examples of advanced isometric exercises:

One-Arm Isometric Push-Ups:

Elevated One-Arm Push-Up Hold: Perform a one-arm push-up with one hand elevated on a platform, hold the lowered position isometrically before pushing back up.

One-Arm Plank: Perform a plank while supporting your body weight on one arm, engaging core and stabilizing muscles intensely.

Handstand Hold Variations:

Wall-Assisted Handstand Hold: Use a wall for support while holding a handstand position, engaging shoulder, arm, and core muscles isometrically.

Freestanding Handstand Hold: Balance in a handstand position without wall support, engaging muscles throughout the body to maintain balance.

Human Flag Progressions:

Vertical Pole Flag Progression: Hold onto a vertical pole and gradually lift legs off the ground, aiming for a horizontal body position, engaging core and arm muscles intensely.

Horizontal Bar Flag Hold: Grip a horizontal bar and gradually extend the body sideways until it's parallel to the ground, engaging core and arm muscles to maintain the position.

These advanced isometric exercises demand exceptional strength, stability, and body control. They're best attempted after mastering foundational exercises and building sufficient strength.

CHAPTER THREE

Isometric Yoga and Flexibility

Isometric yoga poses and isometric stretching techniques can wonderfully complement traditional yoga practices, aiding in building strength and enhancing flexibility. There are ways to integrate isometric elements into yoga and flexibility training, they are:

Isometric Yoga Poses:

Warrior Pose Variations: Hold the Warrior I, II, or III poses isometrically, focusing on engaging and strengthening the muscles while holding the positions.

Chair Pose Hold: Maintain the Chair pose (Utkatasana) for an extended period, engaging leg and core muscles isometrically.

Partner Isometric Stretches:

Partner-Assisted Forward Fold: While seated, partners sit facing each other, legs extended, and gently press against each other's feet to deepen the forward fold, engaging in an isometric stretch.

Partner-Assisted Standing Side Stretch: Partners stand facing each other, holding hands, and gently lean away from each other, engaging in an isometric side stretch.

Isometric Stretching for Flexibility:

Pigeon Pose Isometric Hold: While in the Pigeon pose, engage the muscles around the hip and hold the position, gradually deepening the stretch.

Isometric Splits Training: Lower into a split and hold the position isometrically, engaging the muscles to deepen the stretch over time.

Integrating isometric elements into yoga and stretching routines can enhance muscle engagement, leading to improved flexibility and strength.

Customizing Isometric Workouts

Customizing isometric workouts involves blending them with various training styles to create effective and diverse routines. Here's how you can incorporate isometrics into different training methods:

Combining Isometrics with Other Training Styles:

Strength Training Fusion: Integrate isometric holds between sets of traditional strength exercises. For example, after a set of bicep curls, hold the halfway position isometrically.

Plyometric-Isometric Mix: Alternate between explosive movements (plyometrics) and isometric holds. For instance, combine squat jumps with a pause in the squat position for an isometric hold.

Isometrics in HIIT or Circuit Training:

Isometric Stations in Circuits: Include stations dedicated to isometric exercises within a circuit workout. For instance, rotate between push-up holds, wall sits, and plank variations.

Isometric Intervals in HIIT: Integrate isometric exercises into high-intensity intervals by performing an exercise dynamically for a set time followed by an isometric hold. For example, perform mountain climbers for 30 seconds, then hold a plank for 15 seconds.

By combining isometric exercises with other training styles like strength training, plyometrics, HIIT, or circuits, you create well-rounded workouts that enhance strength, stability, and endurance while adding variety to your routine.

Isometric Training for Specific Goals

Isometric training can be tailored to specific goals, offering benefits for strength building, rehabilitation, endurance, and stability:

Strength Building with Isometrics:

Maximal Contraction Holds: Hold isometric positions at maximum intensity for shorter durations (5-10 seconds) to target fast-twitch muscle fibers, aiding in strength gains.

Progressive Overload: Gradually increase the intensity or duration of isometric holds to challenge muscles and promote strength development.

Isometric Exercises for Rehabilitation:

Low-Impact Strength Building: Isometrics offer a safe way to build strength without putting excessive stress on injured or healing tissues. For instance, isometric leg presses or wall sits for lower body rehabilitation.

Isometric Holds in Range of Motion:
Hold positions within a pain-free range
to aid in joint mobility and muscle
recovery.

**Isometrics for Endurance and
Stability:**

Sustained Isometric Holds: Engage in
longer-duration holds (30 seconds to a
minute) to improve muscular
endurance, such as holding a plank or
wall sit.

Stability Training: Isometric exercises
like single-leg balance holds or stability

ball isometric exercises help improve balance and core stability.

Tailoring isometric exercises to specific goals involves adjusting variables like duration, intensity, and choice of exercises. For strength building, shorter, intense holds work best, while rehabilitation may benefit from gentle yet consistent isometric exercises. Endurance and stability training involve longer holds and focusing on balance-centric movements.

CHAPTER FOUR
Safety and Techniques

Maintaining proper form and considering safety measures are crucial during isometric exercises to prevent injury and maximize effectiveness. Here are some key tips:

Breathing and Form during Isometric Holds:

Breathing Technique: Focus on controlled breathing throughout the hold. Inhale deeply before starting the contraction and exhale steadily during the hold. Avoid holding your breath, as it can increase blood pressure.

Proper Form: Ensure correct body alignment. Maintain a straight spine, engage core muscles, and avoid overarching or rounding your back, which can strain muscles unnecessarily.

Avoiding Overexertion and Injury:

Gradual Progression: Start with shorter holds and gradually increase duration or intensity to prevent overexertion.

Listen to Your Body: If you feel sharp pain or discomfort beyond normal muscle fatigue, stop the exercise. It's essential to distinguish between muscle fatigue and potential injury.

Warm-Up and Cool Down:

Warm-Up: Before engaging in isometric exercises, warm up with light cardio or dynamic stretches to prepare the muscles.

Cool Down: After the workout, perform static stretches to help prevent muscle stiffness.

Proper Equipment and Environment:

Stable Surface: Ensure you have a stable surface to perform the exercises, especially for balance-related isometric movements.

Appropriate Equipment: Use proper equipment, such as yoga mats for floor exercises or resistance bands that match your strength level.

By focusing on breathing, maintaining proper form, gradually increasing intensity, and paying attention to your body's signals, you can minimize the risk of injury during isometric exercises while maximizing their benefits.

Conclusion

The benefits of isometric exercises and how to integrate them into a balanced fitness routine are as follows:

Strength Development: Isometrics build muscle strength without joint movement.

Convenience: Can be done anywhere without equipment.

Improved Stability: Enhances joint stability by strengthening surrounding muscles.

Injury Prevention: Lower risk of injury due to controlled movements.

Time-Efficient: Quick exercises suitable for busy schedules.

Adaptability: Suitable for various fitness levels and easily modifiable.

Incorporating Isometrics into a Balanced Fitness Routine:

Mix with Other Training: Combine isometrics with dynamic exercises, strength training, cardio, and flexibility exercises for a well-rounded routine.

Frequency and Variation: Incorporate isometric exercises 2-3 times a week, varying the exercises and duration for each session.

Warm-Up and Cool Down: Always warm up before and cool down after isometric workouts to prepare and recover muscles.

Progressive Overload: Gradually increase intensity or duration to keep challenging your muscles.

By integrating isometric exercises into a balanced fitness routine and understanding their benefits, you can enhance strength, stability, and overall fitness. Experiment with different exercises, durations, and combinations to find what works best for your goals

and fitness level.

THE END